7 Day Healthy Diabetic-Friendly Meals & Recipes That Wont Raise Blood Sugar

BY Zain ul Abdin

7 Day Breakfast Plan For Diabetics!

Seven-day breakfast plan for diabetics to control your blood sugar and still enjoy their life well for diabetic who want to keep their blood sugar down and don't know what to eat for breakfast and they still want to have a good time right well i have a seven day breakfast plan to get you started hello everyone .

come right now a big egg right they'll only have 70 calories six grams of protein that will be your first day it is calorie efficient protein rich and one egg has less than one gram of carbohydrates right now what if you ate two eggs well if you eat two eggs a day as part of your heart protein diet actually it can lower your fasting blood sugars and your avon sea levels which is an indicator for long-term blood sugar control let's say you're doing that on your first day for eggs it can be cooked poached scrambled and you

can do it in a variety of ways if it is too boring for you can make an omelette with a variety of veggies such as spinach mushrooms bell peppers as an alternative option now because of their high protein and moderate fat and low carbohydrate content eggs are not only delicious but they're ideal for people with diabetes now again you can fry them you know not that fried food is great for you but if it is not affecting your blood sugars occasionally you can do that the second day you go for the yogurt with berries again greek yogurt

with berries is super quick it's nice and pleasant dense choice if you have diabetes now daily products if used in a smart way can actually help regulate your blood sugar levels and even reduce your blood sugar levels right the research shows that and also bacteria in the yogurt which uh help in your digestion and it is great even you know to break down the sugars in your gut which is another finding that in that research that i've seen that the reason that greek yogurt actually helps diabetes with even with

the berries you're getting around very minimal carbohydrates and stuff with yogurt if it is greek yogurt you can do some almonds in there if you want to if you want to have a little bit more calories if you're very active but again you will not have to add a lot of carbs to make it taste good your third day will be chia seed pudding you need to prepare that in advance it is super high in fiber it's beneficial with omega 3s right so chia seeds are super super choice for diabetics for breakfast that's going to be your third day now

those carbohydrates can be absorbed and broken down slowly there are digestible carbohydrates around 12 grams of carbohydrates in one ounce of chia seed pudding but you're getting up to 10 grams of fiber again that fiber has no effect on your blood sugar level because also it slows your digestion and your absorption that soluble fiber in chia seeds may actually help reduce your blood sugar levels greatly i will say a mason jar full of chia seeds for example with some almond milk and vanilla that's your best bet to prepare a nice

overnight pudding with chia seeds all you have to do is refrigerate overnight after mixing it thoroughly calories and the chia seed pudding will be 175 calories around 6 grams will be protein 11 grams of fat and only 16 grams of carbohydrate with a 10 grams of fiber right so if you want to you can actually top the chia seed pudding with some fresh low-carb fruits like blueberries or strawberries for some extra flavor if you like you can use sugar-free sweeteners like stevia for example if you want it sweeter now your fourth day will be oatmeal okay

now that's your fourth day but you are going for the steel cut not the instant ouch okay you are going for a cup not for a bowl they can be healthy if not overdone like if not eating too much because there can still be a carbohydrate load if you're eating too much of it if you're going for half a cup of like cooked oatmeal for example you're gonna need around 250 cc of water to cook that and you're going to end up with 154 calories and you're going to have 5 grams of protein and you're going

to have around 27 grams of carbs in that dish and 4 grams of fiber you know oats help with the cholesterol control as well but there is something in oats it's called a beta glucan that's a special type of fiber again it stimulates a hormone in your gut called peptide yy which you know helps you feel full and that's stimulated by this butter glucon that is present in oatmeal you can add some cinnamon for example some berries some almonds to it or even some greek yogurt if you want to to enhance the

flavor your fifth day will be multigrain avocado on a toast that is simple and is popular you can use a nice multigrain avocado toast that is pretty much suitable for every diabetic as long as you're not eating too many of that now as you know avocados are abundant in fiber and monounsaturated fatty acids which are two nutrients that help keep your blood sugar levels stable after a meal especially breakfast the fiber in the multigrain bread is also a factor so maybe make sure that when you're buying

those you're getting a lot of fiber because some multigrain breads are not necessarily good for you but you are going to end up with you know 30 calories in that and then if you add a half an avocado that will go up to 250 calories 9 grams of protein in that serving 24 grams of carbohydrates and 11 grams of fiber so not bad huh now if you want to boost the protein and fat content in that dish because you're not gonna have a lunch you're going to go for a long time without eating you may throw in there some eggs as well now you put some

pepper and some some salt some chili sauce whatever you want and there you go you have a taste explosion on your sixth day you're going to have a low carb smoothie now yes people can still enjoy a tasty low-carb smoothie and you can have pretty good ingredients in there now even though smoothies are normally having carbohydrates and sugar it is possible actually to make you yourself a low carb smoothie out of a half an avocado half a cup of almond milk and half a cup of greek yogurt and a little bit of a vanilla extract now

more than 254 calories are in there but that's not too bad because you're getting 15 grams of protein 16 grams of fat and only 15 grams of carbs you're getting 7 grams of dietary fiber as well now you can add some stevia if you want some sweetness in there but a half a scoop or a full scoop of protein powder is sometimes also used if you need that extra protein not everybody does some people with chronic kidney disease have problem with that for example but it can help you with the hunger in the long term on the

seventh day you're going to have a fruit and nut bowl with the cottage cheese now cottage cheese i said because it is soft it is creamy it is delicious right and like i said if you use the dairy products your advantage it can actually help lower your insulin resistance which is a super common problem among diabetics right so as a standalone ingredient it is not particularly very tasty or flavorful but if you want it to be even creamier you can actually put in a food processor and blend it you can add some fruits and nuts for example and there you go you have a great sweet delicious ball for your breakfast you are getting around uh in a quarter cup of a cottage cheese you're getting 37 grams of that is with some blueberries for example it's going to contain 190 calories you're going to have 9 grams of protein you're going to have around 9 grams of fat and 13 grams of carbohydrates in most cases and three grams of fiber as well now you're covered don't ask me again what am i gonna have for breakfast for your

diabetes so the seven-day plan and if you keep repeating that it's not boring and it's going to give you results remember that and also remember to subscribe to this channel and also go to our website please and go become a vip member by subscribing to our newsletter at sugarmds.

Easy Diabetic Meals & Recipes That Wont Raise Blood Sugar!

Hello everyone today we are talking about low carb meals that won't spike your blood sugar you're watching sugar md diabetes channel my name is dr ahmed ergen i'm a dermatologist a diabetes educator and a hormone specialist before we get into it especially if you have seen some of our videos and already love them smash the subscribe button right now to avoid missing any content and learn from the expert let's get started i am talking about low carb foods that are quick and easy to make who has time to cook for hours every day

i will first give you some general ideas about how to cook low carb and then in the middle of this video i will give you some specific recipes so stay tuned two things can make the diabetic diet very easy first thing is an air fryer is a great way to cook protein anything from steak to tofu secondly you can cook vegetables in a way that only needs a teaspoon of oil and no extra water because water turns vegetables into mush so i'm not a big fan of recipes that are too long or too complex so they'll make

it easy for you this method of cooking in an airfryer and vegetables make the healthy whole food dinners easy you can use any vegetable or meat in this recipe or recipes but you can basically just change what temperature you cook it at and how long it takes to cook it etc but in my opinion airfryer is a must-have it is not just for making like french fries which you shouldn't eat anyway but airfryer is a really a big part of making low-carb dinners quickly my wife and i cook meat in the airfryer frequently

so why should you buy an air fryer if you don't have one right i'll give you a few reasons number one well it gets really hot much faster than an oven for example secondly it keeps the meat moist while also giving

it a taste that comes straight from the grill number three it is fairly easy to clean and number four around 100 range you can get a good one and i will leave a link in the description of this video below to show you what i like in there and number five it cooks food quickly and number six you don't need to fill up or

stir and if you want to cook vegetables in it you can also do that as well and we use our air fryer almost every day i also don't bother to preheat it because it hasn't been a problem for me or for my wife before if you have an air fryer here are some of the things that we have cooked before and i'll share with you now usually it takes 25 to 30 minutes to bake after the oven has been heated up but it can take longer right uh this is how long the chicken can be cooked in an air fryer depending on how big it is so you can save time from heating up the oven number two it also it doesn't take us to make steaks if you want steaks they always work almost always work out perfectly and you don't even have to fill up the steak to cook in there another thing you can think about is breakfast with turkey sausage or regular sausage but i prefer turkey because i think it's healthier the first thing i do in the morning is to make these especially on the weekends i don't have to be afraid that it will burn on one side etc and often people say basically

just set it and forget it so seriously it only takes four minutes in the airfryer at 400 degrees or 200 degrees celsius uh to cook that food also it goes well with my son's hot dogs as well super easy another thing you can think of is hard boiled eggs can also be cooked in there no need to wait for the water to boil et cetera cook two eggs in the airfryer basket for example for 16 minutes at 250 fahrenheit or 120 degrees celsius for 12 minutes at 300 degrees or 12 minutes at 300 fahrenheit 149 celsius for example

another thing you can think of is tofu if you like the tofu it's time to take the toffee container out of the water if you want to cut soft into cubes you should do so you should also spread out in the airfryer and they should cook for 15 to 20 minutes at 375 fahrenheit around 200 celsius so this will be the best tasting tofu you will ever have okay now with the exception of bacon you can make everything from homemade meatballs to crunchy fried chicken wings and drumsticks to hamburgers and veggie burgers you name it you can even make your own meatballs of course you need to check on your food all you know through the cooking process if it is not done yet just close it again and it will keep cooking for you to your desired temperature now my wife does not cook meat in the oven anymore unless she is making a lot of italian meatballs or something or a thanksgiving turkey and something like that here's another trick for you it is easy to learn how to steam and saute at the same time doing both so when you cook vegetables this way you get the benefit of both steaming and

sauteing right so how do you do that well steaming first of all softens the vegetables without adding any oil and sauteing gives them a crispier touch and a better flavor than just steaming so how do you do that well to start make sure you have a lot of non-running vegetables in your fridge this means that you can buy a lot of these vegetables on a sunday in a farmer's market or something like that or your grocery store and use them all week a lot of vegetables that are in my fridge and we always use a lot of them here are

some examples of these vegetables that you need to have in your fridge all the time celery for example onion beans that have grown into sprouts a great replacement for pasta for example brussels sprout which is a great vegetable and frozen bags work as well and carrots again you can you know buy a bag of pre-sliced if you don't have the time for shopping you know if you live in america everything is pretty much ready to go for you for everything right so that's the cool part of it but you can do zucchini squash uh it's a summer thing but uh green cabbage purple cabbage scallions these are the things that you have to have in your fridge so here's how it works you can put three of these vegetables in a large pan that has a tight lid okay and then follow the steps here so

i can put one or two teaspoons of oil olive oil coconut oil avocado oil etc on top of these vegetables and toss them quickly to make sure the oil is spread evenly around the pan and turn the heat up to medium high like if you're doing a electric one you can do it like a number seven and cover

it with a lid it will be ready around five minutes after that stir the vegetables and cover the pan again when the lid is on the water from the vegetables will be used as a steam source okay now take off the lid after about five to eight minutes or when the vegetables can be pierced with a fork uh steer for another like a couple minutes or so and then decide you know what to do with them the vegetables will be sauteed giving them a crispier look and a better taste at the same time it will be steamed now you can continue to saute

for five more minutes if you want but you know just don't burn it okay um and then you can add your favorite dressing low carb dressing etc or sauce uh salt spices whatever you want to do uh you can do a store bought pre-mixed blend or just salt and pepper will be just fine for some of you now after that half of your plate should be filled with vegetables and the other half should be for your meat that's easy right well we'll talk about more about specific recipes in a minute but you should know that uh sugar md app can

also help you figure out how many carbs you have in your meals so if you don't have our app right now download it at um sugarings.com or just just go to app store and just search for sugar md for both android and for apple

it's more than likely that most of these combinations will have fewer than 20 grams of carbs in total which is great uh but if you're using a lot of green or purple cabbage you know your carbs may start piling up a little bit if you're eating too much of those now how to use herbs and spices well

salty is not as bad as long as you eat whole food and moderation and you do not use like packages on processed foods right the sodium in your food will be mostly from coming from what you put in it and as long as you are using with moderation you should not worry about that too much et cetera unless you're super sensitive with your blood pressure keep in mind that if you're adding a lot of herbs and spices to your vegetables you might want to keep the meat seasoning a little simpler otherwise it'll be too much now another thing to think about is giving your taste buds some time to get used to the taste of the real food if your diet has been mostly processed and packaged foods like if you're used to tv foods these foods may you know taste blend but give yourself some time to start tasting the real food yeah you don't really need a lot of teriyaki sauce to make the broccoli taste good just give some time to understand the real taste of that broccoli again use a flavorful himalayan pink salt for example with other herbs and spices to

help your taste your sense of taste reconnect with the real flavors of vegetables rather than just heavy sauces like ketchup and stuff like that now if you are new to seasonings and start with some of the pre-mixed seasonings in the bacon aisle of the grocery store now some of them may have a small amount of sugar in them but the amount that ends up on your plate will be fairly small a few simple combinations could be for example you can combine paprika and celery you can do salt and thyme and rosemary uh some italian herb blend will

be great or garlic salt you can use parmesan cheese with some salt and celery you can combine paprika with other combinations etc now some of the meat seasoning ideas for you is you can do a dry rub now spices you can basically mix them up and basically rub on the meat right before cooking you can do condiments with a little sugar in them if you want to brush the meat with something before and after so there are a lot of different things you can buy in the store about that as well and number three will be i would say you know just make

your own right to make your own low carb seasoning uh you can basically make some herbs and spices to your taste if you wanna have some aloes to make some sweet taste to

it like the restaurant style that's fine and salt and olive oil you can always brush and sprinkle on your meat before cooking as well it's important to remember that you can use spices in many different ways based on your own taste for instance you can season chicken drumsticks for example or thighs in a bowl and gently press or roll the meat

in a bowl before you put in an air fryer with the desired you know the condiments or spices you can mix slice or cube meat with spices in a bowl as well you can wait until the meat is done or tender before you start cooking them etc

so you can do all sorts of ways now here are some low carb dishes that you should try well you should use the airfryer and the steamer or the steam and saute methods to make a few of my favorite dinner recipes and when you're cooking these recipes always start with the meat first because it takes at the longest time to cook the meat and then move on to other things like your vegetables if you want to cut and saute your vegetables while the meat is cooking great do so there aren't any quantities in this in this recipe that

i'm going to give you because the idea is that you can change the amount to meet your needs and they're simple you don't need to get out like the measuring cups and spoons and ways and stuff like that so it's going to use some simple taste veg veggies and some meat recipes and you'll

be good to go now let's talk about the first one the first one is italian knight well when you're married to an italian that's what you do right you gotta have some italian nights well uh i would say the ingredients will be like turkey based sausage or a regular sausage i prefer turkey over a regular sausage um and the beans that have grown in sprouts sliced onions you can use carrots in small pieces like i said you can buy it in already chopped ones uh perfume giana reggiano cheese remember this

cheese is from the best cheeses video that we have done before so check that out and of course use salt and garlic in that as well now here are the directions in the airfryer put the italian sausage in and of course turn it on if you don't turn it on it's not going to cook right so preheat the oven to 350 fahrenheit or 180 celsius bake about 15 minutes and in order to make sure the sausage is done you can slice one oven and the vegetables should be steamed or sauteed while the meat is cooking now toss the

vegetables with parmesan cheese some salt and garlic salt as soon as everything is done cooking after cutting the sausages you can just basically serve them and enjoy now if you want to cut down on your carbs but still want a side dish i would try a low-carb edamame spaghetti you can find some recipes online about that too now second recipe i'm going to talk about today is chicken thighs and zucchini medley now what are our ingredients in this one well you can use chicken thighs you can do caribbean jerkblend

you can use sliced onion sliced zucchini sliced carrots it is best to apply the caribbean jerk blend to one side of each chicken thai and then you can basically cook the chicken uh that's that easy right and you can do the air fry the chicken thighs for 20 minutes around 375 degrees or 190 celsius and to make a vegetable stir fry put all your vegetables in the pan and cover with the lid and then the food will be steamed and sauteed for you the next on the list is chicken apple sausage and bean sprout medley now the

ingredients for that is chicken sausage and apples of course and sliced onion a bag of bean sprouts some chopped celery and himalayan pink salt you can use parmesan cheese as well in that recipe and slice sausages into bite-size pieces with a sharp knife of course and then airfry should be set at 350 fahrenheit or 180 celsius and you cook it for 15 minutes now in the frying pan you mix the vegetables together and then you can use you can use the uh you can make the vegetables steamed and sauteed as we discussed before

and you can add some himalayan pink salt and parmesan cheese to the vegetables and toast them and mix them up well the next recipe is steak onions and sprouts and yellow squash so the ingredients will be of course steak chopped onions yellow squash uh chopped uh chopped bag of bean sprouts 1 2 teaspoons of olive oil himalayan pink salt and the dressings are going to be um the air frys takes for 15 to 20 minutes at 375 celsius or 190 degrees depending on how you want them cooked you can decide on the time and make small pieces of onion and

yellow squash now pour some olive oil into a frying pan and put the onion and squash and the bean sprouts in in there and then the food is you know just to steam the food and saute as we discussed before and add some himalayan pink salt to the vegetables and and the meat to make them taste wonderful now number five on the recipe is low carb fried chicken no you're gonna be like fried chicken really oh yeah it can be done hear that you're gonna have the ingredients wise the chicken thighs or chicken tenders you're gonna have low

carb flour this could be chickpea flour almond flour or coconut flour you're gonna have um a lot of eggs around 12 eggs and bread crumbs with low carb and then your favorite chopped vegetable combination whatever you like now how do you do that well chicken thighs or tenders should be cut into finger food size pieces before they are cooked and served okay and then fill half of a big zip top bag with some chicken bits shake the bag with half a cup low carb flour until all the chicken is covered and then if you need to add

another egg to the bag and shake it until the chicken is evenly covered you can do that as well and of course you're coating the chicken in a low-carb bread crumbs in this case and then you can basically cook it and serve it now put everything in the basket of the airfryer and turn the machine to cook of course now cook for 20 minutes or so until the meat is done at 350 fahrenheit or 190 celsius degrees while the chicken is cooking make sure you steam and saute your vegetables as we discussed before and then make sure you

make your own dip for the chicken that will be to your taste now as you can see making your own low-carb meals isn't that hard it doesn't take a long time either so if you want to make your food taste better keep a lot of vegetables in the fridge or freezer as well as a lot of a variety of seasonings and some low-carb sauces in your kitchen you just need to mix vegetables and protein sources and then add some tasty spices and use some airfryer that concludes the video guys and ladies if you like these recipes and want to try or already tried it or you have your own recipe you want to share with the community please share in the comment section below so we can all learn and help each other again you just need to mix vegetables with some protein source and then make some tasty foods guys talk to you later stay well hey guys

Nutritionist Cooks Diabetes Friendly Recipes

if you're ready today's episode is about diabetes let's talk about diabetes full name diabetes mellitus common types of diabetes is

type 1.

type 2 gestational and maturity onset diabetes in the young diabetes is essentially inappropriately elevated blood sugar levels

because of lack of insulin or insulin resistance what the heck is insulin insulin is a hormone secreted by your pancreas in the eyelids of langerhan in the beta cells insulin is a hormone that regulates your blood sugar levels just like glucagon you have your meal and what happens is glucose is taken by insulin to be brought to the cells for use now or later so insulin basically brings down your blood sugar levels on the other

hand if your blood sugar levels are too low glucagon will take the stored energy and bring it to the bloodstream to the cells that need it after you eat a meal specifically with carbohydrates this carbohydrate is broken down into glucose

which will then be used for energy either immediately or stored in the liver and the muscle as glycogen now let's talk about the types of diabetes type 1 diabetes is characterized by the destruction of the beta cells in the pancreas like we said that is the cell that creates insulin so basically

insulin has a really hard time being created by those with type 1 diabetes this is often due to genetics and autoimmune in nature so this is the type of Diabetes that usually needs those insulin shots you know

when you see it in the movies they gotta like shoot themselves with some insulin type 2 diabetes on the other hand is when your cells don't respond regularly to insulin otherwise this is called insulin resistance so as much as your body is able to produce insulin it's either your body has a hard time actually responding to it so insulin resistance which means your insulin sensitivity is low and insulin sensitivity is your body's ability to respond to insulin so your body has a hard time responding to insulin even if it keeps on creating as much insulin as possible sometimes the pancreas will start to burn out because it's making so much insulin that the body can't use and the blood sugar levels rise so oftentimes those who have type 2 diabetes are either not producing enough insulin or the insulin that they do produce is not effective insulin

resistance is multifactorial which means there are many possible causes but most often they are from lifestyle factors like sleep diet exercise vices and more but interestingly enough it actually has a higher genetic predisposition than

type 1 diabetes

which means you are more likely to have type 2 diabetes if somebody in your family has it as well Modi on the other hand is a mutation in your Gene which sort of acts like type 2 diabetes but in the younger generations and this is more likely to happen if you

do have somebody in your family who has it as well then you have pre-diabetes so pre-diabetes is you're not really diabetic but your body already exhibits insulin resistance so you do have elevated blood sugar levels oftentimes insulin resistance that keeps on growing over time and not addressed will develop into

type 2 diabetes

next we have gestational diet diabetes so this is the type of Diabetes that occurs in pregnant women who don't previously have diabetes so if you aren't diagnosed with diabetes

and then you get pregnant and then you do develop diabetes this is called gestational diabetes it can often clear up after you give birth but it's usually seen in the second and third trimester of your pregnancy the thing is pregnant women tend to be more insulin resistant because of their extra nutritional needs now that we've gone through the types of diabetes let's ask ourselves what are the signs and symptoms how do I know that I have diabetes or what should I look out for if I should definitely get

tested number one extreme thirst so for example you drink a lot of water throughout the day but even no matter how much you drink you still feel like you are thirsty number two is that constant hunger like we said insulin resistance is

when your body has a hard time actually catching those sugar cells and bringing it for you so your body feels like it's never really fed then we have number three which is constant urination or frequent urination even if you're not drinking that much water you still constantly need to pee then you

have constant exhaustion so your body isn't getting enough of that energy into the cells so you're gonna feel always tired for type 1 you often have weight loss as one of the symptoms well for type 2 diabetes you often have weight gain and in longer cases of diabetes slow wound healing occurs so if you have a wound that is taking so long to heal itself that could also be a major concern if you feel any of these signs and symptoms please consult your physician because because we must get it checked what are the risk factors for

diabetes which means that what are the things that I might have that will increase my chances of having diabetes number one genetics lifestyle factors an unbalanced diet lack of exercise constant overeating these will also increase your risk for diabetes smoking and other vices like drinking alcohol lack of sleep aging unincreased body fat percentage gestational diabetes and also non-alcoholic fatty liver disease I've been diagnosed with diabetes what do I do now well then comes in the management just because you are diagnosed with

diabetes does not mean that it is automatically no hope because there are a lot of ways to manage it you have your lifestyle interventions like working out and shifting your sleep and stress you have your medications and of course your nutritional management do take note that everything we're gonna say here is just a general recommendation

you still need to check with your own physician and dietitian to make sure sure that the recommendations or the plans are made exactly For You especially if you need insulin shots or medication let's first

start off with carbohydrates the feared nutrient carbohydrates are a macronutrient that your body literally needs for energy it's actually your body's preferred energy source especially for your brain and your blood cells what happens is when we eat carbohydrates the body breaks

it down into sugars now sugars is not a bad thing okay this is just what it's called your saccharides so you have glucose fructose and galactose now like we mentioned insulin will be bringing those glucose or those sugar cells to where

they need to go so that they can be used for energy now what we want to do is give your body enough time to process it so that it doesn't feel overloaded so again are carbs bad no the average human needs 45 to 65 percent of their calories to come from carbohydrates so let's dive into our diabetic tips number one choose lower glycemic index carbohydrates again carbs are not bad we just have to choose the ones that can be more beneficial blood sugar wise your glycemic index measures the impact of how fast a food

item will increase your blood sugar and how fast it will drop it glycemic index is higher than 55 usually say that it's probably going to increase your blood sugar a little bit fast while lower than 55 will say that it's going to have a better impact on your blood sugar levels however there is a difference between your glycemic index and your glycemic load and this is often what some people forget or don't give attention to so even if you're choosing your low glycemic index Foods the load or actual

impact to your blood sugar levels will differ for example one piece of bread on its own might increase your blood sugar but to slow it down we can incorporate some fats protein or Fiber like chicken spread or peanut butter that decreases the glycemic load now number two pair your carbs with protein fiber and healthy fats just like we mentioned to reduce your glycemic load you want to pair your carbs or dress your carbs with some companions to slow down digestion and absorption number three space out your carb intake there are some diets

out there that will tell you to just eat one meal a day or just have all of your intake at this time but oftentimes when your meals are just compounded into one time of your day your blood sugar levels can shoot up if you space it out more evenly and equally your blood sugar levels will be much more regulated throughout the day that's why having meals or snacks every two to three hours is often a recommendation by dietitians to their diabetic clients because this can help you manage it better and decrease the risk of complications like

hypoglycemia number four mindful of your fat and salt intake diabetes does focus more on your carbohydrate intake but because it increases the risk of hypertension kidney concerns and a lot of other things we do want to be mindful of the intake that can possibly lead us to increasing other health concerns this doesn't mean that you have to fully change your diet we just have to be more mindful of that intake number five proper energy balance we don't want to eat too much but we also don't want to

eat too little especially because the more you starve yourself the hungrier you get especially since your blood sugar levels will make you feel hungry anyways plus overeating constantly may also Spike that intake but I do want to give a little bit of a disclaimer that there are many reasons why people might struggle with overeating it could be related to restriction it could be related to stress or even the uncontrolled blood sugar so don't be too hard on yourself if you struggle with overeating just be mindful take a step

back and take a look at your overall nutrition and number six lifestyle factors nutrition is one part of diabetes but there are so so many other things that you have to look into your vices your sleep your stress and consistency with your medication nutrition is one part but lifestyle is a bigger one as well so basically that was the breakdown of your nutritional recommendations that was a tough one but don't worry because we're going to apply that into our meals later on in this episode and we'll also be answering some

of your diabetes concerns so let's get cooking let's begin by preparing our onion and garlic did you know that when you crush the garlic that is when the allicin which is the nutrients comes out this always makes me feel the most like professional when I do this and

I was like tada how do we make budget-friendly meals especially when you have to pay for medication you have to pay for doctor's bills and so many things It's always important to know that when you have local ingredients it will always be a

little bit less expensive for example we have malunggay these are ingredients that can be very helpful when it comes to those

who struggle with your budget so this is a very budget-friendly and diabetic friendly dish because it's low glycemic we're using which has a lot a lot of fiber and we're adding as much nutrients as we can can I have rice with my meals how much rice should I be eating how much in general will depend on your overall needs so I can't give an exact amount however I can give a quick tip for those

who like to eat rice but struggle with their blood sugar and that is not to eat hot rice or freshly cooked rice eat it 12 to 24 hours after and

it will have a lower glycemic index with more resistant cervix and now we're gonna add in the mung beans don't forget your water there so while we wait for the to cook as we said we just gotta put it aside it's all good do what you got to do we're also going to prepare our protein and I'm going to be using some tilapia or some fish is fish better than the

other protein sources for diabetes Well it's usually a lower fat source and higher in some and unsaturated fats like your Omega-3s it can be more nutrient dense but it isn't necessarily better you know it doesn't mean that you can only have fish

but it can be a great variety oh salted up and now we pan fry whoa okay we're back to the the fish is cooked and so is the mango so the last thing we add is the malunggay so as we wait for the malunggay to cook I will answer something that somebody always asks me when it comes to diabetes what diet is best for me I'm diabetic is there a specific diet that I should follow generally for diabetics we do a balanced diet with moderate carbohydrates so

 it doesn't have to always be super low carb it doesn't have to be no carb just moderate carbohydrates and we practice carb counting which is making sure that your carbohydrates are well spaced out throughout the day we also prioritize of course your high fiber foods high fiber carbs unsaturated fats so it's more of

like General guidelines and recommendations the Mediterranean diet is often used though for those with diabetes because it tends to follow a lot of nutrition recommendations

it can be very beneficial for diabetics oh look at the malunga it added so much color now it looks like fun to eat yummy delicious all the ingredients are ready let's plate it so we have our brown rice here nice high fiber lower glycemic index and then we have our so now we're going to put it in the bowl and just like that we've got a meal

let's jump into making our snacks so we're gonna make like an egg wrap so we're going to be using our egg as a wrap for this dish is there any specific fruit or veggie or is there anything that is very specific for diabetics as long as you are eating them in their full form rather than juice because that's where most of the fiber will be definitely up to you what you will choose but when it comes to fruit it will depend on the amount per serving so fruits do have fiber but we don't want to have like a giant bowl of mangoes at

once it would be better to spread it out throughout the day one of the questions that we got in the previous episode the one on Picos and diabetes asked us the question of can we differentiate type 1 and type 2 diabetes so they're actually very different and that is actually why we made a whole episode dedicated to diabetes because it's still completely different from Picos although they do have some similarities so Ashley mentioned in the beginning of the episode type 1 diabetes is usually autoimmune in nature a destruction of

the beta cells in your pancreas giving you a hard time or your body can no longer produce insulin which is needed to use the carbohydrates well type 2 diabetes you're insulin resistant which means you're able to still produce insulin in some amount

but you're not as efficient as at using it diet wise there aren't major differences it's just that you have to be a little bit more aware of your insulin shots and when you take your insulin if you have type 1 versus type 2. it just means that when you're

type 1 diabetic

the difference is really trying to time it with your medication for those meals and also being aware of your blood sugar levels throughout the day that's why you see people taking their blood sugar in between the meals or in between the day so they can really watch it so we're gonna flip and pray at the same time that's it

let's finish up our wrap now put our ingredients on top so our question is on gaining weight while diabetic so if you're underweight and you're trying to

gain weight with diabetes how do you do it without raising your blood sugar levels it's also important to note that in these situations it's very important to consult with your dietitian because you have to know if you're **type 1 diabetic type 2 diabetic** any other health concerns that might need a little bit more intervention

but generally it's about increasing your calorie intake and if you are struggling with increasing your blood sugar per meal then spreading it out would be important and also again

incorporating your higher calorie food items that aren't too high in carbohydrates but of course if you are type 1 diabetic because it's common for those who have type 1 to lose weight then it would be a mixture of having a dietitian on board to help you out and your medication so these are all General recommendations you still need to consult for your own specific case okay it's time to taste our dishes I'm excited and this is actually the one I'm excited for so we'll start with this one

um taste healthy but it's good it's a fish it rounds out the whole dish I think this is going to be really filling really satisfying high fiber perfect okay let's move on to this one everybody's waiting for this one this is like a crap I'm gonna Savory crap but a little bit of sweetness from the Greek yogurt wow I did good well and there you go two really easy and when I mean easy I mean easy because I have literally no skills in the kitchen so this is doable for anybody out there high fiber moderate carbohydrate very helpful for those with diabetes

DIABETICS Must Be Eating THESE 11 Best Breakfast Foods DAILY!

Did you know that one in every 10 people in America suffers from diabetes?

Time and time again, we have been reminded of the importance of breakfast. Typically, it consists of toast or cereal. However, choosing the right foods can be quite a task for diabetics.

Having the right food to power through the day is important. A balanced diabetic-friendly breakfast   consists of lean protein, fiber, healthy fats and non-starchy vegetables. This also means replacing regular, everyday breakfast foods with low sugar   alternatives. Wondering which foods to choose? Greek yogurt with fruits? Oatmeal with berries? Avocado with fried eggs?   Today we will talk about breakfast foods for diabetics.

Avocado with Fried Eggs Let's start off with a popular breakfast choice you may have seen on social media. Avocado paired   with fried eggs in the form of a salad or on top of a sandwich is not only deliciously filling,   it's packed with nutrients that will help stabilize blood sugar levels.

The good fats   and omega 3 fatty acids of avocado combines well with the lean protein of fried eggs to create a   power-packed breakfast meal. They also help reduce inflammation, adding fiber and heart-healthy   minerals. The best part? You can get creative with the seasoning and add the herbs of your choice.

What's your favorite avocado toast topping?   Sound off in the comment section and start   a conversation with our Bestie community! Hummus with Whole Grain Toast When it comes to breakfast for diabetics, you have to think outside the box.

Hummus, which ranks extremely low in the glycemic index, is often overlooked. However,   it can be a saving grace for them, as it's a healthier alternative. Hummus is made by mashing   chickpeas into a smooth, butter-like consistency and mixing it with some garlic and salt.   Consisting of minimal ingredients, it's light, but still packs quite a punch.

Just spread some   hummus on top of whole grain toast and sprinkle some chia seeds on top for extra nutrition. Roasted Vegetable Egg Omelet Vegetables and egg omelets are two really filling meals. Instead of just having a plain old egg,   add some veggies! Mixing veggies adds tons of nutrients to the otherwise traditional egg.

But how does it help in maintaining glucose levels?   The roasted vegetables contain fiber that contributes to the slowed digestion of food,   resulting in a much more stable blood sugar level. Eggs also constitute for healthy protein   while the veggies are a source   of various vitamins like K and C.

Omelettes are already healthy. Adding some roasted vegetables like tomatoes, broccoli, carrot and spinach to it will add more nutritional value, and make it a more balanced   meal. Delicious in taste, packed with nutrients and wholesome, this omelette is easy to whip up. Oatmeal with Nut Butter A bowl of oatmeal may sound basic, but that's not the case.

Diabetic or not, it's a great breakfast   option for everyone! Who doesn't want to start their day feeling full and active? A wholesome bowl of oatmeal topped off with organic nut butter will keep you active throughout the day.   The soluble fiber that is packed in oats not just lowers cholesterol levels and protects heart   health, but also reduces glucose absorption.

This means that the fasting blood sugar tends   to remain stabilized. The combination of oatmeal and nut butter improves digestion   and fills up on antioxidants, which will improve your skin and hair. Grilled Peanut Butter and   Strawberry Jelly Sandwich Eating sweets is an absolute no-go for people with diabetes.

But not anymore! Starting your   day on a sweet note just got sweeter! Organic   sugar-free peanut butter on wholewheat bread, topped off with a small amount of strawberry jam is the perfect recipe for your breakfast.

The base, being made of whole grains, contains a good amount of fiber that slows the breakdown of   food. The peanut butter layer gives you a ton of nutrients including vitamins, calcium, manganese and much more. The jelly is simply to add some taste while keeping the blood sugar level stable.   This combination of foods, when eaten together, creates a healthy diabetic friendly meal.

Berry Smoothie Looking for a time-saver? Mixing up a berry smoothie is a nutritious and delicious way of   kickstarting the day. Blackberry, blueberry, strawberry and raspberry are known for their awesome health benefits. It keeps you mentally sharp with nutrients called anthocyanins.   A glass full of berries is loaded with antioxidants that increases immunity and gets rid   of toxins in the body.

When it comes to diabetes, this smoothie also fights off inflammation, a major contributor towards diabetes. To pack some extra nutritional value and make it extra-filling,   add some unsweetened greek yogurt, banana, and a little spinach. Drink up! Sweet Potato Hash Sweet potato fries are huge! Sweet potato hash is also a healthy alternative to the regular potato   hash. Being low on the glycemic index, eating it guarantees no rise in your blood sugar level.

The orange color is because of the presence of carotenoids,   known for lowering the risk of developing cancer! You can eat it as a side dish for your breakfast   or substitute it with your favorite potato dish for a healthier version. You can prepare it easily   by combining grated sweet potato with delicious herbs and spices, and then baking it in an oven.

Whole Grain Cereal Eating cereal while living with diabetes is not a good idea. Sure, it's very cheap,   quick to prepare and requires no recipe whatsoever.   Regular cereal contains large amounts of sugar, which are bad for blood sugar levels. Whole   grain cereals contain rich amounts of fiber and   protein without unhealthy artificial sweetener.

Replacing regular flour with whole grain will lower the risk of stroke and other   heart related problems. If losing a few pounds is your goal, regular workouts is the secret   along with switching to whole grains. To add texture to a whole grain cereal,   you can add pumpkin seeds, flax seeds or coconut shavings! Thinking about replacing flour bread? Here are the 5 healthiest types of bread to eat.

Now back to diabetic friendly breakfast foods. Chia Seed Pudding The saying 'don't judge a book by it's cover' applies to chia seeds. These gluten free, vegan friendly seeds are a perfect addition to your breakfast.   Not only do they add an earthy, nutty flavor to water, puddings and salads, they also keep   the stomach full until it's time for lunch.

 Chia seed pudding is the perfect healthy breakfast meal loaded with omega 3 fatty acids, fiber, protein and is a favorite among vegans. These nutritionally dense seeds have a positive   effect on glucose levels since it promotes a   slow release of carbohydrates. This means that the fasting blood sugar remains stable   while filling the body with nutrients you need to stay active through the day.

Pumpkin Quinoa Berry Bowl It's no doubt that quinoa is the ultimate breakfast food for diabetics. The complex carbs   with fiber and protein are slowly digested, which doesn't cause any crazy changes in blood glucose. Another reason to make it your breakfast is that you won't feel famished by mid-morning.

Pair it up with mashed pumpkin and berries of your choice! Pumpkin also provides essential nutrients like carotenoids, vitamins C & E and folate,   all of which help strengthen the immune system. Adding berries,   nuts and seeds will elevate the nutritional value of your breakfast and make it even more filling.

Eggs and Lentils on toast Eggs have always been regarded as a superstar breakfast food. Diabetic or not, they're the go-to choice for a quick, healthy breakfast. However, just eggs are not enough, you need something else to balance out, not just the taste, but the nutritional value.   Although lentils are not one of the most famous choices for breakfast, they have good reason   to be among the top choices.

Lentils are   an immediate source of fiber and protein,   two ingredients needed to build muscles and stay lean. Inexpensive and prepared quickly, eggs, lentils and toast will quickly become your favorite breakfast. Breakfast has to be one of the most neglected foods in the world.   People either ignore it or don't devote much time into preparing it.   Skipping breakfast is not an option for diabetes patients.

To make the most of your eating habits,   a diabetic also needs to adopt a healthy and active lifestyle.

10 Best Foods Diabetes Type 2 Patients SHOULD Eat DAILY | Diabetes Diet Food and Snack List

10 Foods People With Type 2 Diabetes Should Eat Daily Diabetes is a chronic disorder that affects the way the body metabolizes sugar. It is caused by two problems: 1) The pancreas doesn't produce enough insulin, or the insulin it produces doesn't work correctly. 2) The cells in the body don't respond properly to insulin.

Diabetics are at higher risk of developing heart disease, blindness, and nerve damage. Therefore, it is essential to make sure they are eating the right foods to keep their blood sugar in check.

A healthy diet for diabetics should consist of good carbs, fats, and healthy proteins but in small portions. People with type 2 diabetes are generally recommended to consume no more than 1,500 to 1,800 calories per day.

Diabetics also need to make sure not to overeat since it can raise their blood sugar levels. The following are some of the healthy food options that diabetics should eat daily: 1. Olive oil There is a big misconception that if you have type 2 diabetes, you cannot have any fats in your diet. This is false because unsaturated fats are essential for a person with type 2 diabetes.

Trans and saturated fats are the ones to stay away from because they can promote weight gain and increase heart disease risks. Extra virgin olive oil is known for being one of the "good fats,"

but it also contains other healthy nutrients important to the body. It is rich in monounsaturated fats, which studies have shown can help lower "bad" LDL cholesterol levels.

Extra virgin olive oil also contains antioxidants, which can help reduce oxidative stress in the body. This means that it can act as an anti-aging agent by fighting free radicals and reducing oxidative stress. It can also prevent cardiovascular disease and cancer. 2. Nuts & Seeds Frequent nut and seed consumption can reduce the risk of developing type 2 diabetes.

This is because they are high in fiber, protein, and healthy fats, which can help control blood sugar levels. Nuts and seeds, when eaten in moderation, can protect people with diabetes from developing serious complications. However, it is important to note that people with diabetes should limit the portion size because they are high in calories.

3. Eggs Eggs and other protein-rich foods can be an important part of a diet for people with diabetes. They can help regulate blood sugar levels and prevent severe spikes in the short term. Eggs are also rich in vitamins and minerals, including antioxidants lutein & zeaxanthin, which can help prevent diseases related to the eye.

Each egg only contains 80 calories. 4. Peanut Butter To help control blood sugar levels, experts recommend adding some healthy carbs to your diet. Some people find that peanut butter is an excellent substitute for refined carbohydrates like white bread and sugar. These people find that the energy from the peanut butter lasts longer than the quick burst of energy from refined carbs.

However, it would help to watch how much peanut butter you eat and your salt intake because too much salt can cause high blood pressure and other health problems. 5. Green Vegetables People with diabetes should increase their intake of green vegetables like spinach, cabbage, or kale, to reduce their risk of developing complications associated with diabetes.

Furthermore, studies have shown that people who eat green vegetables regularly are less likely to get type 2 diabetes or develop complications from it. 6. Cinnamon Cinnamon can be used in various dishes for flavor, but it also has some health benefits. Some research has found that cinnamon can improve insulin sensitivity and reduce blood sugar levels in people who have type 2 diabetes.

03:47

If you're interested in taking cinnamon supplements or adding it to your food, be sure to use Ceylon cinnamon instead of Cassia cinnamon. Ceylon has more health benefits and fewer unpleasant side effects. 7. Dark Chocolate Dark chocolate has many health benefits that can help people with diabetes. Dark chocolate is high in antioxidants, which can help to reduce free radicals in the body and combat inflammation.

This means it may help to reduce the risk of cardiovascular disease and protect against stroke or heart attack. It also has a higher cocoa content than milk chocolate, which studies have shown to improve blood sugar control for people with type 2 diabetes after eating. 8. Beans and lentils Beans and lentils have a low glycemic index, meaning they release their sugars into the bloodstream slower than most other foods.

They also have a high fiber content with both soluble and insoluble fiber, which can help lower blood sugar levels by slowing down digestion, reducing the absorption of sugar from the gut, and increasing feelings of fullness. In addition to lowering blood sugar levels, beans and lentils are also packed with protein that can help those who suffer from insulin resistance or those on diabetic 9.

Brown rice Brown rice is a whole grain that provides fiber and some vitamins and minerals. White rice is a refined grain that has fiber and many minerals removed, making it softer. Brown rice is healthier in many ways, but people should still keep their carbohydrate intake in moderation to avoid weight gain.

10. Avocado Avocado contains monounsaturated fatty acids, which are good for managing blood sugar levels and insulin resistance. It's also full of fiber and antioxidants that help keep your body healthy and fit. A research study shows that people who eat half an avocado with lunch or dinner for 12 weeks can lose more weight than those who don't add avocados to their meal plan.

That's a roundup of some foods for diabetics to eat daily to maintain a healthy lifestyle and take care of their diabetes.

9 Fruits You Should Be Eating And 8 You Shouldn't If You Are Diabetic

Did you know that 11% of the American population has diabetesBeing a diabetic is a difficult job. You have to control what you eat along with getting ample amounts of exercise. Diabetic or not, for a balanced diet it is important to eat fruit every day. Contrary to popular belief there are some fruits that contain unhealthy amounts of sugar which cause a spike in blood sugar levels.

Finding a diabetes-friendly fruit that can help keep your blood sugar in a healthy range is difficult. Is there a way? Here are the best and worst fruits to eat if you have diabetes. Are peaches and apples good? No more pineapple and banana? Stay tuned to learn everything about the good and bad fruits for diabetes.

Let's start off with the best fruits! Blueberries

 Blueberries are superfoods for diabetics. These tiny tangy fruits are packed with vitamins, essential minerals and tons of antioxidants. Not only does it promote overall health, it also gets rid of free radicals. For long term diabetics, eating a bowl of purple salad, containing blueberries, purple cabbage and feta cheese, will help in increasing insulin sensitivity and glucose processing.

Blueberries ,strawberries or any other berries in general, are a diabetic's best friend. With a glycemic index of 53, you can add these miracle berries to parfaits and yogurts as well. A refreshing way to start the day! How do you like blueberries? In a salad? Power juice? Tell us in the comments!

Peaches

Peaches define the summer season. They are a super healthy addition to your daily diet, low in calories, are a wonderful source of fiber, potassium and vitamins A and C. It is the perfect fruity treat for diabetics to satisfy sweet tooth cravings and help with weight loss. Peach smoothies or salad, it's up to you! The antioxidants and vitamin C content help in fighting off free radicals and makes your skin and hair look healthier and softer.

Apricots

Apricots' sweet flavor, and impressive nutrient content, makes them a worthwhile addition to your diet. They come loaded with beneficial vitamin A, C, potassium, copper and manganese. Eating dried and whole fresh apricots help in maintaining blood sugar levels. Unlike commercial sweets and chocolate that contain sugar and processed carbohydrates.

For a healthy diet having it thinly sliced with peanut butter toast is a wholesome meal for diabetics. Their low glycemic index and nutrient content help regulate diabetes. They also improve digestion while making the body feel full. Apple Having an apple a day may keep the doctor away. For diabetics - keeping a tab on carb intake is key.

You may think that apples contain carbs, but the fiber in them helps in neutralising this effect and maintains the blood sugar levels. A medium sized apple contains around 25 grams of carbs. The fiber content is about 4 grams. That helps slow down the digestion process and very slowly releases the glucose in the bloodstream. It's good news for diabetics!

Oranges

When you think about an orange you think, Vitamin C and citrus but it's more than that! Citrus fruits like grapefruit, lemons, limes and oranges also contain Vitamin A and iron. The nutrients in them reduces inflammation, the possibility of cell damage and also protects the heart.

The folate and potassium helps in controlling diabetes. Packed with fiber and a low GI index, they're also one of those rare fruits that gets slowly released into the bloodstream. Remember to get the best benefits out of oranges or any fruits, it's better to eat it whole rather than drink the juice. Kiwi Kiwi is a great choice for diabetics.

Not only is it delicious, it's also rich in antioxidants. With the focus being improving immunity these days, it is also a great way of keeping your immune system healthy. This is due to the presence of free radicals that destroy any toxins present in the body. Kiwi keeps heart health at its best! With a GI index of 53 it stands in the lower ranks, making it the perfect addition to a diabetic meal plan.

Pear

Pears can be very tasty and are a great fruit to eat if you have diabetes. Their nutritional benefits can actually help you manage the condition. They also have a low glycemic index,

so they won't raise your blood glucose too quickly. As long as you keep your portions in mind and eat them along with other nutritious foods you should go for it! They are dense in nutrients and vitamins that have several health benefits like fighting inflammation and helping with digestion.

Remember to always eat a whole pear with the skin on because most of its nutritional goodness comes from the fruit jacket. Cherry Cherries are more than just a delightful cake topping. When eaten in the right manner, they have some incredible health benefits. One cup of cherries has 52 calories and about 12 grams of carbs, which has inflammation fighting properties.

Did you know that they also contain melatonin that helps you get a sound sleep. When it comes to blood sugar, they have diabetic goodness as well. Although small in size they are packed with antioxidants and are low in the GI index, which plays a significant role in maintaining blood sugar. Along with all of these benefits, they also protect heart health.

Thinking about making some tweaks in your diet? Then check out this video: "9 food combinations that will benefit your health" and make meal prep a breeze. Now back to the best and worst fruits for diabetics. Strawberries Did you know that 1 cup of strawberries contains more Vitamin C than a whole orange? These delicious berries have a very low GI index and are totally safe for diabetics.

Strawberries have several good nutrients like antioxidants, fiber and Vitamin C. Berries in general, like blackberries and blueberries, are perfect to kill those sweet tooth cravings. They are also known for their detox properties which keeps your immune system strong. Now - let's see fruits that all diabetics should avoid: Pineapple Pineapples are considered one of the healthiest fruits on the planet.

Packed with Vitamin C, manganese and antioxidants, they are a great way of staying healthy. Sadly, they are not pleasant news for diabetics. Ranking extremely high on the GI index, pineapples contain gross amounts of sugar that cause exponential spikes in blood sugar. If you still wish to enjoy this amazing fruit, then make sure to eat it with foods low in carbohydrates.

Watch your total carbohydrate intake for a wholesome, balanced, diabetic diet. Mango Often referred to as the 'king of fruits' this tropical delight is a no-go for diabetics. Mangoes are loaded with a variety of essential vitamins and minerals, making them a nutritious addition to almost any diet. But they also contain loads of calories, sugar and carbs which is another common culprit in increasing blood sugar.

If you still wish to enjoy a mango smoothie or slices then remember to go for firm mangos rather than the pulpy ones. Watermelon Watermelons contain several health benefits and a variety of minerals and nutrients. These range from Vitamin A, B and C to folate, fiber and magnesium. Along with hydrating you they're loaded with antioxidants and contain lots of sugar.

Although present in natural form, if eaten in large quantities watermelon will spike blood sugar levels. With a GI index of 72 it should either be eaten in moderation or completely avoided. Banana A banana is an excellent choice of fruit for your morning breakfast. It helps you stay active throughout the day.

Although healthy for everyone else, diabetics should avoid them! Bananas contain high levels of carbs, sugar and calories. Eating it causes a rapid increase in blood sugar. Although it contains fiber, diabetics are advised not to eat it because even a medium sized banana contains 14 grams of sugar.

Grapes

Grapes are a good way of getting in some vital nutrients like Vitamin C, K and essential fiber.

They help in boosting the immune system, are the perfect food for the brain and make your hair and skin look healthier. A cup of grapes contains around 23 grams of sugar which is unpleasant news for all diabetics. Popping a couple of them may seem innocent but can cause serious trouble if not kept on check.

Raisins

Raisins are sweets that have become a superfood recently. They contain loads of antioxidants, are low in calories and have fiber that makes you feel fuller for longer. Unfortunately, they're a no go for diabetics. They contain large amounts of sugar, even though it is a healthy snack they contain carbs that get converted into sugar when released in the bloodstream.

Try to keep your raisin intake in check or just enjoy them in moderation. Lychees Lychee is a good source of vitamin C, potassium, copper and manganese. Plus are a good source of fiber which comes in handy for losing weight. Sugar is present in every fruit but the type of sugar present in lychee is different and may cause harm to people with diabetes.

It is also not a good choice for people with gestational diabetes because every piece contains a whopping 29 grams of sugar. Dates Over the years dates have become one of the most popular alternatives for sugar. Due to their sticky nature, dates are also used as a binding factor for homemade granola bars.

Being dried and processed, they are highly concentrated with calories and sugar. Just 1/4th cup of dates have 100 calories. If you don't have your diabetes under control, avoiding dates is the best way to go. Which fruits didn't make the cut? How do you deal with diabetes? Share your tips in the comments!

18 Healthy Diabetic-Friendly Snacks You Should Be Eating

Snacking often gets a bad rep, but if you are managing type 2 diabetes, including healthy snacks in your diet can be a great way to keep your blood sugar levels balanced and energy levels up Choosing healthy snacks can be difficult when you have diabetes.

The key is to pick snacks that are high in fibre, protein and healthy fats, all while keeping your blood sugar in mind. In today's video, we will tell you the best snacks for diabetics. From almonds, popcorn, organic beet chips, egg muffins to black olives and more, watch till the end to learn about all of them. S

imple Guacamole: Simple...but filling, this guacamole can be savored with crunchy cucumber slices to keep carbs in check. Plus, the polyunsaturated fatty acids found in avocados are known to improve insulin making it easier for the body to regulate blood sugar levels. Just peel and chop avocados, then place in a small bowl. Sprinkle with lemon juice. Add salsa and salt. Now mash coarsely with a fork and refrigerate.

What's your favourite snack to go with guacamole? Is it raw vegetables? Nachos? Or something else? Tell us quickly down below in the comments section! Sugar-Free Hot Cocoa Made With Dark Chocolate: Sip a warm cup of sugar-free hot cocoa to beat the munchies.

One cup of fat-free milk blended with   one envelope of sugar-free cocoa mix scratches that chocolate craving. It also gives you about 400 milligrams of calcium, nearly 30 percent of your daily value of this bone-building mineral. Look for a sugar-free dark-chocolate cocoa mix because dark chocolate offers   more benefits than the milk chocolate or white variety.

Popcorn: Popcorn is the king of comfort food. But did you know that it's a whole grain, too?   Whole grains contain satiating fiber, which can support healthy weight goals. This high-fiber,   crunchy snack tantalizes the taste buds. But be mindful of what you put on top.

 Select a low-fat variety of popcorn   that can be microwaved or air-popped for   just 6 g of carbs and 31 calories per cup. Edamame: Cooked edamame provides roughly 17g protein and 8g fiber in one cup. This is why it's considered a powerful snack for keeping hunger levels in check.   This diabetes-friendly munchie is available fresh or frozen, so it's super easy to make.

Plus, the bioactive compounds in these   beans are also known to protect heart   health in multiple ways such as lowering cholesterol and reducing blood pressure. Mini Babybel Cheese: For an on-the-go snack that   will fill you up without impacting blood sugar levels, try Mini Babybel Cheese.   This fun snack is 100% real cheese and a good source of calcium and protein.

Since it contains 0 grams of carbohydrates, you know your blood sugar levels will stay   within a healthy range even after your snack. Pair it with a handful of raw,   non-starchy vegetables such as sliced red, yellow, or orange peppers, baby tomatoes or   sliced cucumbers. This will add volume, vitamins, and minerals without extra carbs or calories.

Oatmeal With Berries: Who says oatmeal is   just for breakfast? A study found that eating   it for just two days helped diabetics get their blood sugar back on target. One ½ cup of plain, cooked oatmeal contains 77 calories,   3 grams protein and 14 grams of carbohydrates.

Quick-cook oats are high on the glycemic index   while steel-cut ones are a better choice for people with diabetes. Top your bowl with ¼ cup of your favorite berries — such as blueberries, strawberries,   or raspberries — as well as a ½ oz of almonds. This will fill you   up and keep blood sugar levels stable for under 200 calories. Spicy Pumpkin Seeds: With 7 grams of protein per ounce, pumpkin seeds can help squash hunger in minutes. These seeds are also a great alternative if you have a nut allergy.

Studies suggest that   this festive snack can slow down the absorption of carbs in the gut keeping blood sugar balanced. Consider adding plain, shelled varieties to other dishes such as salads and baked goods. They're also high in magnesium, a mineral known to protect heart health. Rhythm Organic Beet Chips: These beets have all the spectacular crunch of potato chips,   and they include far more beneficial nutrients.

These simple, conveniently   packaged beet chips are ready to snack on. Just reach into the bag to start crunching. The beets have been dried, so they won't make your fingers all red, but they still have all the good stuff like fiber and iron. The snacks are USDA organic and non-GMO Project Verified,   and they are healthy enough to snack on any time, or even all day long.

Celery sticks with hummus: Celery is a low-calorie, high-fiber food that also provides   vitamins and minerals. Pair it with hummus to add a source of protein. For best results,   avoid highly processed hummus, and make it at home by blending chickpeas, tahini, and lemon.

Chia seed pudding: Chia seeds are a great superfood.

They are rich in protein,   omega-3 fatty acids and fibre. They can prove extremely effective in managing blood   sugar and are remarkably easy to add to your diet. To prepare chia seed pudding, take 3 tbsps of chia seeds and mix with 1 cup of almond milk.   You can pick the milk of your choice.

 Although this step is optional,   you can add 1 tsp of honey and mix well to sweeten it. Leave the   mixture in the fridge overnight and top it with fruit before you eat it. Egg muffins: Eggs are one of the best sources of protein,   and are very fulfilling as well. This makes them diabetes friendly. Mix and bake them   with vegetables or the meat of your choice and you have got yourself a delicious snack.

To prepare, preheat the oven to 350 Fahrenheit, spray oil over the muffin tray. Take 5 eggs,   chopped onions, pepper, salt, and a half cup of cheddar cheese and whisk . Divide   the mixture into the muffin tray and bake   it in the oven for at least 20 minutes. Eggs are beneficial for your body in more ways than one.

To know what we are talking about,   watch this video titled "This Happens To Your Body When You Eat Eggs" Now back to healthy snacks if you are a diabetic. No-bake energy balls with cinnamon: Made from high-fiber oatmeal, peanut butter, crushed walnuts, and banana, these bars have   about 12 grams of carbs and 4 grams of protein per ball. They have no added sugar.

Walnuts are   another great source of healthy omega-3 fats that help reduce inflammation and protect the heart. Combine 2 cups rolled oats, 1 cup peanut butter, 1 cup crushed walnuts, and 1 tablespoon honey in the bowl of a stand mixer.

Beat until well combined, adding more honey if the mixture is not holding together. Using a cookie scoop, form 20–24 balls and place them on a cookie sheet. Dust with cinnamon powder. Refrigerate for 30–60 minutes or until firm. Unsweetened Greek yogurt with berries: Greek yogurt provides gut-healthy probiotics and a good amount of protein. A single-serving contains 14 grams of protein and only 6 grams of carbs.

Be sure to buy unsweetened yogurt since some flavored ones contain as much as 20 grams of added sugar per serving. It's best to skip the brands with artificial sweeteners as well. Sweeten yogurt with a handful of berries, which also provide filling fiber and inflammation-fighting antioxidants.

Black olives: If you love savory foods but want to steer clear of junk, try a single-serving pack of olives. While olives are often criticized for their high sodium content, the high fat content of these fruits comes from monounsaturated fat, a powerhouse of the Mediterranean diet. Because they're already pre-packed, you can easily watch your portion size.

Fresh, Low fat Mozzarella and Juicy Tomatoes: Fresh mozzarella and tomato is another good choice of snack for diabetics. When it comes to cheese, it is recommended to eat reduced-fat or regular cheese in small amounts. One oz of fresh   mozzarella supplies 6 grams protein and 6 grams fat. One cup of grape tomatoes has 8 g of carbs.

Skip the dressing and opt for a drizzle of heart-healthy olive oil or balsamic   vinegar and a dash of salt and pepper for flavor. In total, this snack is about 130 calories. Almonds: Research suggests that a handful of almonds just might keep blood sugar stable.   Thanks to the naturally present fiber, protein and healthy fats.

With a perfect crunch, this   shelf-stable snack is ready whenever and wherever you are. Getting bored of plain   varieties? Explore your spice rack and splash on some exciting seasonings to create Spicy Almonds. Cantaloupe and Creamy Cottage Cheese: Low-fat and low-sodium cottage cheese enhances the natural   sweetness of cantaloupe. Top 1 cup of cut-up melon with ¼ cup of low-fat cottage cheese.

The melon is an excellent source of vitamins A and C. Plus,   the low-fat cottage cheese adds 7 g of protein to the snack and supplies a good source of calcium. Add a sprig of mint to add a punch of color and flavor. A small apple with peanut butter: Yes, this   childhood favorite is diabetes-approved.

Apples are high in fiber with the skin on, low in calories, and rich in flavonoids that   may be protective against diabetes. Peanut butter offers some protein and healthy fat,   but cap your serving to one tablespoon if you're aiming for a lower-calorie snack. While these are some great snack ideas, it's equally important to eat the right   food all the time if you're a diabetic.

Get to know what foods we're talking about by: Finding out foods diabetics should be eating Or Learning about fruits you should be eating and ones you shouldn't If you are diabetic These 2 videos will definitely help expand your meal options if you're   diabetic. Do you prefer healthy or unhealthy snacks? Let us know in the comments below!